AF712906

Table Of Contents

Introduction: You Will Survive.

I know it doesn't seem like it.

But our team is here to tell you that you will.

As the mountains of books, lectures, handouts, quizzes and tests begin to pile up it certainly feels like a death sentence.

But it's not.

Like most of us who made it into med school you are an intelligent, hardworking, and a dedicated student. All those hours spent with your nose in the biology and organic chemistry books will finally pay off as you realize, "Damn, I really can study." Inside yourself you'll find the grit that you need to make it through. I promise.

Medical school has often been described as trying to drink from a fire hydrant. Personally, we can't think of a better metaphor. The sheer volume of information that you'll be exposed to is unimaginable. Even though you will be saturated with information, there will also be an overriding sense that you are missing all the important stuff. To make matters worse, this is only a small fraction of the medical knowledge that exists today, all of which you will be expected to master over the course of your career. A recent quote reminds us that the sum of medical knowledge doubles every 73 days.[1] As a doctor you will be expected to keep up with all this material, and medical school can help prepare you for this inevitability.

Being a doctor is fun, interesting, challenging, discouraging, and heartbreaking. The first year of medical school will attempt to prepare you for this by slamming so much content into your brain that you'll feel like your head will explode. It may seem asinine and downright insane, but this method helps build your resilience for the future. By the end of your first year, you will be a master at collecting and organizing information in your head, memorizing things you once thought impossible, and regurgitating vast amounts of information in an intelligent and appropriate way. The Kreb's cycle will become second nature. Complicated biochemical pathways will become child's play. Your mind will literally be at its peak performance. Most importantly, you will realize that while the grades are nice, they aren't nearly as important as learning and understanding how to be an amazing physician and take great care of your patients.

The easy answer is to just power through, head down, maybe taking brief pauses to complain about the difficult hours and time required. However, first year of medical school offers you an incredible opportunity to grow as much as you learn, and our suggestion is that you enjoy it while it lasts. For many people, medical school will be the hardest thing you've done this far (residency may be harder, but you aren't there yet – don't worry about it). The most important lessons you learn during medical school are not from the lectures but the long hours and hard work that teach you about yourself, add iron to your bones, and grit to your step. Many physicians will relate to the feeling that

How To Survive Medical School Year 1

Mark Wiseman & Missy Desouza

With Jessica Barkhouse, Alisha Tillman, and Jonathan Bishop

Angela Karulak and DM Kashmer, Editors

MARK WISEMAN & MISSY DESOUZA

HOW TO SURVIVE MEDICAL SCHOOL YEAR 1

Tips, Tricks, & Stories From Survivors

"the smartest I've ever been was at the end of my second year in medical school." It may not seem like it now, but this is one of the defining points in your life. Take a moment and breathe it in.

Know that you, my friend, are reaching the very pinnacle of academia and learning. Like those adventurers climbing to the peak of Everest you will push yourself to a new level that many find impossible.

The most important thing to remember is you will survive. The pain and agony are only temporary. You will come out the other end. When you do, you will be surprised at just how much you have learned along the way.

In this book, you will hear from various voices and perspectives. We did our best to make this personable and relatable. We wanted to tell our own stories so that you can feel the truth and validity behind them. While much of the book is written as combination of our voices and experience, we wanted to give the true sense of two separate perspectives. Therefore, any section that comes from a particular individual will show their name in italics beforehand.

We hope that by reading this book we can spare you some of the agony that we experienced, having been through the pain of medical school and learned most of our lessons the hard way. We assembled this book together in an effort to condense what we've learned into one cohesive platform. Make no mistake, medical school will still be quite painful, hopefully with this book you can learn from our mistakes and have a more pleasant experience.

Stick with it. Stay strong. You've got this.

Chapter 1: Grit, Determination, and Alcohol.

Section 1 – Make a Schedule Already

Many medical schools differ in the way they approach lectures. The majority still offer good old-fashioned sit-down lectures where boring (did I say boring? I meant extremely engaging and interesting...ahem) professors tell you everything you need to know. However, more and more schools are transitioning to an online curriculum, where all the content is delivered via pre-recorded lectures. While this may seem incredibly convenient, and it is, it makes scheduling and organizing your time even more important.

We can't tell you how many times we heard a friend tell us they were going to be up for the next week straight catching up on lectures and videos. This strategy might have worked for all you crammers in high school and college, but all-nighters like this will likely have you running out of steam quickly. Take, for example, this medical school experience from our team...

The first year was infamous for a period of time in February and early March where students were given 48 (yes, 48) exams within a two-month period. For those of you doing the math, that's an exam every other day. If you were to try and do an overnight cram session for all that madness, you literally wouldn't sleep for a month. You may have evolved or been constructed to function without sleep, but the rest of us *Homo sapiens* need some sort of rest.

Our recommendation is to set up a schedule. Imagine that studying is your job: you should put in about eight to ten hours a day. Think this is a lot? Well then, you're going to be sorely disappointed when you find out that this is a breeze compared to residency, when you're expected to work 12-16 hour shifts and then go home and study. Compared to that, 8-10 hours a day is a breeze!

Your schedule doesn't have to be all studying at once. In fact, research shows that humans learn better if they study in bursts.[2] Study for about 2-3 hours then build in a break for yourself. Go to the store, get your shopping done, go to the gym (yes, go), walk outside, then get back to it.

Speaking of the gym, we can't stress enough the importance of regular exercise. We're not talking about becoming a world-class athlete here, but you need to keep your mind and body healthy. The best way to accomplish this is with about 45 minutes of exercise 3-4 times a week. This amount of exercise has been proven to improve cognitive function and endurance. The small sacrifice in time here will pay off in truckloads when you are sharper and more engaged at one in the morning studying for your microbiology final.

With the amount of volume thrown at you in medical school, sticking to a schedule is vital. It will help you stay on top of topics and not get behind. Falling behind in medical school is nearly a death sentence, as the sheer amount of information can be impossible to catch up on. More so, if you can make a schedule and keep it, you will be pleasantly surprised by how much you accomplish. You will retain more and be less stressed come exam time.

Mark: This was literally my one and only secret during my first year. I constantly had people coming up to me asking me how I knew so much and how I was doing so well. My answer was simple: I put in the time and made a reasonable schedule. I treated every day like a work day and didn't let myself deviate. This was probably the number one reason for my success during first year, so I recommend it to anyone and everyone starting out!

The next thing is something you probably already know. In the modern age, everyone is trying to come up with ways to improve education and understand how humans learn. From this research, the understanding of different learning styles has evolved.[3] While it might seem trivial, knowing and understanding your learning style can be essential to performing well. Find out what things work for your early. Do you need visual stimulation? Are you a reader? Do you do better if things are said out loud? This can alter your study methods immensely. Look around online and take a test to get a sense of your learning style!

Mark: Personally, I was (and still am) a very visual person. I would spend hours drawing out my anatomy and physiology, knowing that once it was drawn out it would be cemented in my head. This also meant that I spent a lot less time listening over lectures as I knew the information wouldn't stick as well. I also found that flash cards were amazing as they provided me a visual stimulus while getting the background info, plus it was something I could do while watching TV or some other activity.

When it comes to time management skills, there's nothing like multiplying your time. This is a strategy implemented by many CEOs and businessmen and women. It essentially means finding ways to do two or three things at once. Can you read while running on the treadmill? Call your mom while reviewing your pharmacology notes? Find ways to do the things you want while studying at the same time. Flash cards are a great example, but be innovative and find ways to learn while doing things you enjoy. There's only so much time in the day, and medical school will constantly have you wishing for more hours. The more you can integrate your study and life schedule, the easier it will be.

As you're planning your days, don't forget to factor in that some activities have a high brain demand and others have a low brain demand. For example, studying is high, but buying your groceries is low. You are human and cannot study 24/7 as much as you may think you can. Your brain will get so fried that you can't get any high-quality studying done (and slamming your head against your books in frustration, hoping that some information seeps in doesn't work, trust us). There's no point wasting your time on low-quality studying – you've got to take a break. And these breaks are the perfect time to incorporate in those low-brain demand, mundane, essential activities like laundry, groceries, cooking, or cleaning.

It may seem like those things are trivial compared to the all-important task of studying, but the truth of the matter is you'll feel better if you do them. There's something about waking up to a clean room, having clean clothes to put on, and eating a nice meal that makes you think, "I've got it together, I can do this." It signals to yourself (and to others) that you're in control and doing just fine. You'll perform better in school, build your confidence, and build your professional persona if you can keep all that up.

Don't let the temptation to slack off get the better of you. As said before, medical school is crazy! To quote our school's Dean, each semester of medical school is equivalent to taking 45 college-level credits worth of classes a semester. Compare this to the normal student's 10-18 credit load. It's pure insanity, which is why we recommend you be equally insane. You must be crazy about your work and crazy about your schedule (let's be honest, you're already a little bit crazy for applying to medical school in the first place).

Also, don't get discouraged or distracted by the people who seem to work less than you do. As said before, everybody will have to work hard in medical school, brilliant or not. For some people it will come easier, while some are just better at pretending. As with all of life, you will always find someone who does something better than you do or seems to not need to try. Keep working and keep your schedule, find your own ways of doing things and discover your strengths and weaknesses. Only you know you, so don't look elsewhere for all the answers.

Mark: You may see some people appear to not have to work at all (see: my frustratingly brilliant co-author). Don't fall into this trap! Chances are this isn't you. I myself made the mistake about halfway through medical school of assuming that I could only put in part of the effort and do as well as some of my more brilliant colleges. I was wrong. I learned the hard way that my success was a result of my grit and discipline. If you are anything like me, this will be true for you as well. Don't let those annoyingly smart people distract or frustrate you! You got into medical school on your own, and you're smart and tough enough to make it through, just stick with it!

Missy: Mark freely calls me annoyingly smart, but he is probably why I made it through medical school as successfully as I did. Because concepts came easily to me, I was NOT great at setting a study schedule. As a result, when some tough life events set me back at the beginning of my second year, I didn't know how to catch up. Mark helped me set a schedule and stick to it (more or less) to prep for the endless exams. Part of working smarter is to identify your shortcomings and build workarounds to keep you on task. Use your strengths to your advantage and enlist your friends to keep you on track!

Tips and Tricks from Recent Survivors:

- Schedule your breaks. If you don't schedule your breaks in, you won't ever take one. Scheduling time for yourself also helps diminish the guilt you feel for taking a break and not studying. For some reason, medical students believe they are superhuman and don't need rest, but we definitely do. Feeling guilt about not studying is normal but not something you should succumb to.

- Establish a sleep schedule. When you have to decide between working through a couple more lectures or getting that extra hour of shut-eye, it can be incredibly tempting to sacrifice your sleep for the sake of productivity. Sacrificing your sleep is almost always the wrong choice. You've got to be rested if you want to have high-quality study time, so make sure that you get minimum of 6 hours of sleep a night. Figure out when you study best and build your sleep schedule around that. It's okay to stay up till 2 a.m. studying if you wake up at 9 every day – and if you are a night owl this may result in better studying! Whatever times you decide, start to develop a routine around that so you don't fall into the trap of skimping on sleep.
- Low-brain demand times: Friday afternoons, after exams, during the afternoon sump – these are all great times to do all the chores you need to do. Also, grocery pick up is a lifesaver for cutting down on the time (and money!) you spend shopping.
- Declutter your brain space. All the small decisions in your life can add up. If you find that you are wasting energy making decisions about your outfits or breakfast, then streamline those decisions to save your thinking for things that matter – like school.
- Have a place where you can keep on top of hardcore deadlines and exams. We found the easiest way to do this is an old school calendar/planner, though there are a plethora of apps that you can use as well.

Section 2 — The Transition

You might think you're prepared, but you're not. The transition from college to medical school is one that knocks even the most brilliant minds flat on their back. While it's true that there are certain individuals who can put in less effort than you and still succeed, there is a limit. Unlike college where certain people could sleep through lecture and still pass, there is no one that escapes medical school without having worked their ass clean off. Even our most brilliant friends still found themselves stuck in the library for hours memorizing long lists of information prior to an exam.

The trick is not to let yourself be overwhelmed or scared in the beginning. For most, the first few months of medical school is like a tidal wave: you are constantly being bombarded with an impossible amount of information to learn and integrate.

One of our good mutual friends came up with an excellent analogy. Imagine you are a new Ikea employee. Your boss comes to you with a stack of Ikea manuals and says, "I need you to read these and memorize them. Tomorrow you'll get another set. At the end of each week I want you to be able to assemble every item from memory." You do this, every week, for the next two years. Medical school is like that.

We don't mean this to frighten you off, but a little bit of healthy anxiety can motivate you to come in prepared and ready to face the challenges that will be put in front of you.

Some medical schools attempt to give you a slow transition while others force you to hit the ground running. Either way, you'll find that once you're in the thick of things, as long as you keep your head and stick to your plan, the rest will come. One of the most amazing things about being human is our adaptability, which becomes even more evident after a few months in medical school. Your brain will get used to being bombarded with information and you'll become even more efficient at learning and processing.

Just as with high-level athletes, you need time to get in shape. You need training. The initial period (in fact all of first year) can be considered pre-season. You'll be subjected to the hardest workouts and training so that by the time the game comes, it'll seem like a cake walk. Your brain adapts much the way your muscles do. The more you work it and train it, the easier each workout becomes.

This means you need to give yourself some credit and leeway in the beginning. Give your brain time to adapt. Don't be frustrated if you feel overwhelmed. This is normal. It will come with time, just be patient.

Make sure to overcompensate that first week of school. The worst thing you can do is fall behind. If you are grinding hard through those first tests, you can always slow down for the rest of the block. But it is really hard if you didn't do well in the beginning to kick it into a high gear half-way through.

Another useful strategy would be to find an older student who has already been through the process to help guide you. Many medical schools provide a mentorship program. If your medical school does, definitely take advantage of it. These people who have been through the ringer and survived can provide you invaluable tips and tricks for surviving and even mastering the different subjects. Older students are invaluable because they can give you access to resources that people have compiled for your school, old study guides for hard professors, and tips & tricks to get through. However, make sure during the first few weeks that you don't get so caught up listening to everyone's advice that you sacrifice your own studying. Older students will always have a plethora of advice and will want to tell you all the things they learned that worked for them that is the "best" way to study. Listen to them, but don't hold their word as gospel. You still need to decide what works best for you personally.

As you meet people at school, especially early as students are still transitioning in, there can be a lot of insecurities and anxiety. Most everyone who has made it to medical school was considered one of the smart kids in college. It can be an unwanted shock that first week when you sit down in a class full of geniuses and realize you aren't as special as you thought. A lot of people compensate by talking loudly and proudly about impressive research they did in undergrad, their copious hours of volunteering, and a myriad of other achievements that will make you feel like you don't compare. Most of these are overinflated. Most of the people who feel the need to subtly flex about their accomplishments are the most insecure. Don't be like them. Deal with your insecurities in a different way.

On the other hand, identify and address imposter syndrome early. Imposter syndrome is a term to describe the feeling that you don't belong, and that maybe it's a mistake that you're in medical school. It can be an incredibly isolating and crippling frame of mind if you let yourself think that way.

Here is the truth that will help you avoid imposter syndrome: you may not be the smartest kid in the class any longer, and maybe you were never the smartest kid to begin with; but if you are in medical school, *you are smart*. If you've made it this far, you're meant to be here. You deserve to be here. Don't let anybody tell you otherwise.

Section 3 – Alcohol. Sweet, Sweet Alcohol.

Missy: I'm going to put it right out there. This chapter is about blowing off steam, not necessarily about drinking. While we found alcohol played a significant role in the relaxation methods of our fellow medical students, there are other ways to let loose. There are also many pitfalls to overindulgence that can cut short your medical career before it has even started. Work hard, play hard, but responsibly (mostly).

One of the most important parts of medical school is NOT the work, it's about giving yourself enough rest to succeed. Continuing with the athlete analogy, through decades of research we've found now that one of the most important pieces to athletic training is *rest*.

As your body experiences stress, it triggers pathways that initiate rebuilding and growth. If you continue to stress the body, these pathways run out of energy and can't function. However, if you give yourself enough time to recuperate, these pathways will add the strength and endurance required to meet the challenges you face.

This is the same when it comes to learning and your brain. You may not realize it now, but your brain can get fatigued (oh boy, you will learn this soon). As you consistently tax your brain's resources, it runs out of energy and needs to be repleted. It may be tempting at times to simply drink the pain away and go party, but a better and healthier option is to let yourself sleep, relax, get exercise, and enjoy some downtime.

Recent research into neuroplasticity has demonstrated that your brain is constantly being remodeled and rebuilt. Which means that you still have the ability to rebuild your brain in the way you want (sounds like something out of a bad sci-fi movie). This also means you need to provide your brain with the proper building blocks as well as the time needed to make the changes.

One of the emerging ways to give your brain the rest it needs is through mindfulness meditation. It may seem hokey at first, but a lot of my colleagues and attendings have adopted this practice with great benefits. A lot of modern research has shown benefits of meditation. Take the time, give yourself a break, and find a good mentor. For many, this seems to be the most effective way to reset yourself. [4]

Or... you could do what the rest of us do and drink a lot. Like a whole lot.

Mark: Work hard play hard is the motto, and the majority of us stick to it. I'm pretty confident in saying that most of us have been at our most inebriated the nights following some gigantic exam. I would tell you about the amazing party we had after our anatomy exam, but I still don't remember it...

Going out and drinking with friends is often a fun way to get rid of stress. As always, be safe. All things in life should be done in moderation. At this point you probably already know the downside to excessive alcohol consumption. You'll probably have to face an awkward conversation with that one classmate the next day. Be prepared for the worst hangovers of your life as you get older and your metabolism can't catch up.

And, in all seriousness, be on the lookout for true alcoholism.

During our time in med school most of us probably qualified as binge alcoholics. However, there was this one friend who truly was, and dealt with it.

Deacon (don't assume that's his real name), a close friend, a great person, and an even better surgeon, came into medical school with the mentality that he had in college – to drink the town dry and spend whatever leftover brainpower he had on school. While being brilliant and able to skate by half the time, even he found out that this would catch up with him.

During small group exercises, he often would be found lying under the table trying to milk his hangover (yes, this really happened). Charismatic and always friendly, it was easy to go along with his antics and laugh it off. However, as with most of these things, it eventually caught up with him.

During one of our final projects where we had to prepare an hour-long case report, Deacon had done his normal routine and stayed out until four the morning drinking. He showed up to the presentation with alcohol on his breath and a fresh cowlick on his head. Normally able to play this off, he was startled when he bombed the presentation, as the teacher could clearly see through his friendly demeanor. Fortunately for him, she made the choice to sit him down and confront him about his habits. Deacon still relates how this was a turning point in his life, and that he realized that his college ways of drinking and not giving a damn would no longer work. Without this intervention, Deacon admits he might have ended up in a gutter somewhere.

We share this so that you don't have to suffer the same experience. Alcohol can be a wonderful way to shed yourself of the social boundaries that keep you restrained, but, as with everything, understand the dangers. You are about to embark on one of the most difficult and stressful endeavors of your life, and the temptation will be there. Be mindful of it and overcome it.

Tips and Tricks from Recent Survivors:

- Find a way to play hard and do school the next day. It isn't always practical to go out drinking every time you need to let off steam. Find a way to decompress with your people in a constructive way. We found that group sports, "family" dinners, and game nights were a great way to hang out with your classmates and have a good time but still be able to wake up and study in the morning.

- You can't play hard if you're always talking about school. When you're with your classmates, it's hard to talk about anything else other than the one thing you all have in common: school. Avoid this trap. We made a rule that if you were caught talking about school when we were out, you were publicly shamed (and sometimes forced to take a shot). It made our down time a lot more fun.

Section 4 – I'm Not Crazy, You're Crazy

The discussion about alcohol abuse and its sequelae allows a perfect transition into our next topic: mental health. While it is often a taboo topic that people don't or won't talk about, we promise you it is essential. Mental health is more than just as subject matters for your boards. You are about to be pushed to the brink of your mental capacity. While some deal with this with lots of alcohol and guns (yes, guns), others deal with it by becoming wholly and completely depressed.

While true depression is its own monster to be understood and dealt with, the majority of the people we were friends with and interacted with at some point in time felt depressed or anxious. The sheer stress of impending exams can drive any normal person out of their mind. So, it's important to acknowledge this and deal with it early on. In Medicine, we are trained to be adept problem solvers. **But the eye cannot see what the mind does not know**, so you can't solve an issue with your own mental health without identifying it first.

We personally recommend seeking professional assistance through some sort of therapist or counselor early. While it may seem trivial at first, we guarantee that after you only scored a 97 on your first anatomy exam and you're crying in the basement in the micro lab (ahem, what? Never happened) that this person will feel like a godsend. Everyone needs someone to vent to, especially in times of extreme stress and pressure, and having a blank slate in the form of a mental health professional is invaluable. Many programs have counselors on staff exclusively for medical students for this purpose. Seek help early and often while you still have some degree of control.

If you're still not convinced, then this is where the importance of a good network of supportive and understanding friends comes in. This doesn't have to be friends in medical school, although this does help as they tend to be in the same boat. This can be friends from home, good friends from college, or simply family. One of our mutual friends in medical school could be found in the front lawn, on the phone, crying to her mother after every exam (she got honors, by the way).

If you do find yourself truly depressed or anxious, don't be afraid to seek the help that you need. A bout of anhedonia from depression can be crippling to your study schedule, let alone to your personal life. Everyone knows that medical school is one of the most difficult and demanding endeavors one can undertake, asking for a little bit of help is not a weakness. Find the help that you need and get yourself on track. You'll thank us later.

Tips & Tricks From Recent Survivors:

- If you have any inkling towards anxiety or depression, medical school will bring it out of you. That's okay. It has become increasingly acceptable to be on low doses of medications for this during medical school and then taper off as you find you need it less. The important thing is to recognize when you start developing these symptoms and address them early.

- If you find yourself functioning fine at school, but developing anxiety or depression any time things start slowing down (on break or during slow weeks), you may be suppressing your emotions and thoughts to help you survive school. Don't overlook this sneaky manifestation of mental illness – it is still an indicator that you are not functioning at your peak!

- Quality over quantity applies to your studies, and in order to have high-quality studying, you must be self-aware of your mental state. Understanding when you're are not in the right head space is important so you can reset, decompress and get back to efficiently studying at a high level again.

Chapter 2 – Never trust Anyone Named Meredith

Just like when you started college, medical school throws you into a completely new social environment with a completely new group of people. This means entirely new possibilities: friends, enemies, and general annoyances. While it can be tempting to just be friends with everyone, experience has taught us to be a little bit more selective with relationships.

Mark: As an example, I'll tell you a story of mine. I started medical school with the mindset that friends were a distraction; I believed that all I needed was me, myself and I. Obviously this mindset is inherently flawed. Medicine as a practice is dependent on people being able to work with each other and trust each other. One of the most important skills you can learn early on is how to interact with your future colleges. I see far too many people ignoring this and thinking they can take on the challenge on their own. You can't, it's too big.

I digress. Well, a few months into my first year I decided that it would be worthwhile to make a few friends. One of the first friends I created, largely out of convenience, was a girl named Meredith. She was friendly enough and appreciated when I would help her or talk to her. She also seemed to have a good heart and would always talk about how she wanted to help people. Wow can looks be deceiving. About two months into our friendship, I began to suspect that something was awry. She began to belittle me in minor ways and talk down to me when doing certain tasks. She also wouldn't let me out of her sight. More so, she insisted that I help her study, saying that she needed my help to succeed and that since I was doing so well it was my responsibility to help her with her work.

This culminated in a single drunken night (remember how I warned you about alcohol??) where things got a little too friendly. Nothing major, but more than I had expected. However, I woke to a stream of angry texts telling me that I had destroyed the trust between us as friends and required repentance in the form of doing her most recent assignment. Yes, I kid you not.

Fortunately for myself at this point I wizened up the fact that I was being taken for a ride. While the intentions may have started out pure, clearly, I was being used as a way to improve school, not as a friend. This person then went on to be just as crazy as I suspected, and I learned to be careful about the friends I choose.

(Believe it or not, I found out years later that Meredith had spent the first six months of medical school telling our classmates that her and I had been dating and physical on the regular, neither of which were true in the slightest. This goes to show that the medical school application process weeds out the weak, but not the crazy.)

What's the moral of this tale? To be careful with whom you give your trust. Unfortunately, medical school happens to attract very intelligent and ambitious people but does a poor job of selecting out those who might be malicious. We call them gunners: those who would be willing to throw your sorry carcass under the bus so they look better. They exist in droves in medical school, and can make your life miserable, so the best bet is to avoid them at all costs.

While it may be tempting to find the socialite in the group, often these people won't be the best person when action comes to studying and succeeding. Sometimes that nerd hiding in the corner that you never would've spoken to in college is actually the most valuable person to make friends with. Find the people who will protect you when you make a mistake and will stay up with you all night studying when the going gets rough.

Tips & Tricks From Recent Survivors

- There is enough to go around. If you are constantly jumping on every research project, conference, and leadership position that you hear about, your colleagues will avoid telling you about them. It means a lot to hear, "I heard about this awesome opportunity and thought you'd be a great fit for it." If you are the person finding opportunities and sharing the wealth, people will start running to you when they hear Dr. Whoever is looking for someone to research that thing that you love.

- Don't be a gatekeeper. When it comes to school, the biggest competition is yourself not your classmates. You will only benefit from sharing freely with others.

- Distinguish between friends and colleagues. You should be kind, respectful, and helpful to everyone in your class, but you don't need to be best friends with everyone. You need to be selective with who you invest your energy.

- If your school still has grades, don't compare them. Your grades shouldn't be other people's business or a topic of discussion. Even if you have friends who you feel comfortable discussing grades with, don't do it in places where other students can hear you. If you hear people talking loudly about grades in class, avoid them. Those are red flags for bad friendships.

Section 5 – Avengers, Assemble!

Just as important as it is to find and avoid those individuals who would suck your lifeblood, you need to find your core crew of co-studiers. As stated previously, everyone has their own learning style and their own strengths and weaknesses. One thing that medical school teaches you is that even the smartest, most aggravatingly brilliant people have limits.

You *will* be better than someone at something. It might be interacting with people and making friends. It might be pharmacology. It might be psychiatry. Hell, it might just be drawing (we're looking at you, JLee). Whatever it is, find it and use it.

The first part of this emphasizes something we already discussed: find your own superpower. Find what it is that you're good at. Discover your learning style, how you approach problems, and what allows you to organize information. Once you've done this, you can find a group of people whose strengths complement yours.

> *Mark: My experience says that each person typically has a single best subject. Don't be shy, if you find the one that you excel at be proud of it and use it to your advantage. For one, this will give you some insight into your learning style. Secondly, it gives you some bargaining power. Say, for example (ahem... may or may not be exactly what I did) ... that you are a very visual learner and excel at anatomy, however can't wrap your brain around all the names required for pharmacology. Well, you can now convince your oh so pleasant colleague who happens to be a names wizard to help you with pharmacology while you walk them through every body part. Multiple times. Over and over again.*
>
> *Not to be underestimated, I myself was blown away during board prep when one of my co-med students literally couldn't figure out what the parts of the elbow joint were. Seriously. Yikes.... but then she went on to totally destroy me in pathophysiology (and now is an amazing cardiology fellow in New York).*

The beauty of Medicine is that it allows for a wide variety of people with an even wider variety of skills to all work in the same field and find their niche. No two people are going to share the same strengths. This will only become more obvious as your career in Medicine progresses. You might as well take the time and take advantage of this early on, as it will be a part of your career for the rest of your life.

In the meantime, we recommend that you form your own Justice League. Find a group of individuals that you can trust, that are tolerable to study with for hours on end, and whose skills complement each other. Take advantage of the time that you have and learn from the other brilliant people around you. Who knows, you might just end up being friends after all is said and done.

Tips & Tricks From Recent Survivors:

- You may need to change who you study with based on what subject you are studying. You may find that the subjects that are more memorization heavy (Pharmacology, Microbiology, etc.) lend yourself to studying better with certain people. However, those same people may not be the best people for you to study understanding based classes (like Physiology, Pathology, Anatomy, etc.). It is okay to switch up study partners as you feel the need.

- Laugh a lot. Medical school is full of studying, tears, and long nights. The least you can do is try to smile and laugh through some of it. Part of the joy of studying in a group is all the fun you get to have with them.

- Celebrate victories and losses with your groups instead of playing the comparison game. When people in your group are struggling, stay that extra hour to help them through another couple lectures. When they finally pass that test, buy them a drink and treat it like they won the Olympics.

- Be open minded to alternate ways of studying. There is no point in having a study group if you are so proud that you can't accept their help. If you find yourself leading the study sessions in every single topic, you may not be open minded.

Section 6 – Find Your Friends

In an ideal world, your study partners will be your friends, but that's not always the case. And that's ok.

Mark: One of my closest and most valued friends was my roommate during medical school and we never once studied together. Not once. This was probably mainly because we would distract each other with the latest South Park episode or argue who the hottest professor was. But we were able to recognize this and find other individuals who allowed us to focus and succeed when working.

One of the mistakes I made coming into medical school was believing that I didn't need friends to get through. I thought that I only needed a series of business partners and study comrades, so I would be wholly focused on school without distractions. This turned out to be a mistake, as without the support I needed I found myself burnt out quickly. If it wasn't for the friends I had (somewhat accidentally) made, my career in medicine could have easily been cut short.

The truth is that medical school is the equivalent of four years of boot camp. You will be tested mentally and emotionally. It's important to have a support system of people going through the same thing in order to push you through the stress and anxiety. Thinking back almost every single one of us had a breakdown at some point, and it was in those times that we relied on our friends the most to bring us back.

Just like boot camp or getting deployed, there is a level of isolation that comes with medical school. Many people are moving somewhere new to start school, but even if you have family close by, they rarely understand what you are going through. You can easily lose track of what is happening in your family and friend's lives because you are trying to survive what you're doing right now. In the midst of the loneliness that can ensue, your friends from medical school can come and support you along the way and serve as a reminder that you aren't doing this alone.

Much like with soldiers going to war, there's a level of camaraderie that you reach when going through a stressful environment together. These individuals with whom you are facing medical school with will likely become your brothers and sisters through fire. Some of the strongest bonds of friendship we've ever made were in medical school, and we contribute it to the ordeal that we went through together.

Mark: My best example of this was my friend John Lee. Both brilliant and friendly, both of us attributed our success during our first year to each other. Halfway through the first year we discovered that our learning style was similar. We thus would spend hours and hours before tests writing out complicated biochemical pathways and reiterating frustratingly difficult physiologic systems to each other. Both of us would routinely say that it was this last bit of studying and reviewing that allowed us to fully understand the material. It was also during this late night and long hours studying that we developed a solid friendship that would last forever. John saw me during more than one of my meltdowns prior to the exam, and never judged me for it. Being in the same boat and going through the same hell together, we could understand each other on a deeper level than most. To this day we still keep in contact with each other, even though our careers have sent us on very different directions.

Chapter 3: Dating in Medical School. Don't.

Section 7 – Good Luck

The truth is that the experience with dating in medical school is quite varied, which is why we made this section with multiple perspectives. Having drastically different experiences in medical school gave us very different perspectives.

The problem is the same in any situation: *you have no free time*. While this might seem simpler when you're single, in fact in makes it very difficult to find the companionship (and let's be honest, sex) that you're craving on your worst days. It can be very hard to find a significant other (or friend with benefits) willing to put up with your schedule that often prevents you from talking to, seeing, or even acknowledging them.

Part of the trick, as with everything, will be finding a way to efficiently schedule them into your life. For the most part, if you can establish a pre-agreed upon arrangement for time it will make things go smoother. You should make it clear far ahead of time that you will not be as around as other significant others, and that this is something they will need to accept. In addition, they need to understand that at least for the next four years school comes first.

Not everyone is ok with accepting this. If you choose to power forward, be prepared for difficulty. We personally recommend that you try to focus on people that do understand. But if you choose otherwise, know that things will be difficult. Many people expect a significant other to be around to comfort and console them. They want to have a partner that can experience life with them.

During this period of time, you will be limited. This is something you will need to reiterate time and time again.

Coming in with a pre-existing relationship is difficult enough, but it becomes even more difficult when you are trying to break into the dating scene while you're in school. Some of our friends found this a great way to blow off steam and get away from all the school talk for a minute. Others found this emotionally draining and time consuming.

No matter what camp you fall in, don't feel bad for what you choose to do. There can be pressure from both sides on whether you should be dating or not. People might give you a hard time for spending all your energy on dating when you could be doing school instead. From the other side, there is the never-ending pressure to get a move on and find the one before you get old and cranky.

Ultimately, medical school is just school and shouldn't have the final bearing on whether you date or not. After first year, you'll be busy studying for boards, then busy doing rotations, then busy with residency, then busy with a job. Don't let the business of all this make decisions for your personal life and values. If you want to date, go date! You will be able to make time for it, but it will just require a little more finesse and sacrifice.

Section 8 – For The Women: All The Single Ladies

The single life in medical school is, well, different from all your prior experiences. While many programs are in cities, your new schedule basically guarantees that your social life will turn into that of a Tibetan monk, possibly with similar hygiene habits (awesome for attracting potential hook-ups). Happy hours and social engagements come at the expense of sleep and grades. Regardless, there has to be some way to have it all. I mean, everyone on *Grey's Anatomy* is banging it out in call rooms all over the hospital and they're *RESIDENTS* and must be way busier than medical students, right?

If shows like that teach you anything, it's that while you may not have as much time to go out to meet people, you will be working in close quarters with plenty of attractive, intelligent, and driven people. Most of these people are very relationship worthy and could help your career. However, you will be spending a disproportionate amount of time with your med school classmates, and let's be honest, these are not socially well-rounded, emotionally mature, ex-supermodel humanitarians.

During your time in Medicine, you will inevitably meet a resident or doctor who met his or her spouse in medical school and are living the American dream with their 2.5 children and labradoodle. In fact, two of our good friends met during their first year, were fortunate enough to stay together through match (more on that in later years), had a beautiful and fabulous wedding (complete with raucous afterparty), and now live in enviable relationship bliss in Philadelphia (with said doodle). But going by the odds this is probably not you.

The hardest part about trying to date a classmate is that med school is smaller than college. A lot smaller. So, if things don't go well after a poorly timed alcohol-fueled adventure post week-one mixer, you will have to face that person, every day, in the hallway for the next four years. Also, I hate to admit it, but your classmates talk. Since no one else has a social life, if you have one it will be the talk of the class, and people with either try to live vicariously through you or bring you down.

The next part of dating in med school is the double standard. there are two levels to this 1) guys v. girls, and 2) single v. professional.

Missy: If you're female, I'm sorry, but dating is going to suck compared to your male counterparts. Your profession affords you zero game at bars. Women may literally throw themselves at your male classmates who drop hints that they will be a doctor, no matter their other shortcomings. Nurses will try to date them, or set them up with other nurses, or invite them to orgies (yes, that happened).

As a female, you will instead get asked how nursing school is going or asked if you are trying to get your "Mrs." degree. In all reality, the people who are threatened by a strong female are not the kind of people you want to get involved with in the first place, but that doesn't make them less annoying. As a female, my advice to the guys in med school is to definitely play the future doctor card if you want to get laid and don't care about consequences.

Talking about consequences brings us to 2) single v. professional. This goes back to just how small medical school can be and how much people talk. If people know you are dating, they will talk about it. If people know you hooked up with X, they will talk about that. If X is a classmate, then your professors may even know it.

Regardless of if you are male or female, your sexual exploits with be talked about with equal fervor and you will be judged on surprisingly equal footing for your, ahem, frequency of activity and variety of partners. The fact is that everyone is sexually frustrated, no one has enough time to do anything about it, and that leads to a lot of angst.

We thought we graduated from high school drama. What are you doing here?

Missy: The key to keeping it professional is don't talk about it. If you are responsible, make safe sex choices, get tested (Microbiology will make you fear all human interaction ever), and engage in consensual adult relationships with your partners, the gossip gods smile kindly upon you. If you brag, pick the wrong partners, get caught out on the walk of shame, treat your partners poorly, or ask the residents on rotation to prescribe Plan B for you (yep, also happened), then be prepared for a smiting with the slut stick.

We could name the trashiest people from medical school, and they weren't always the ones who always slept with the most people, just the ones who were the most vocal about it.

There are ways to be publicly and very actively single without a chorus of haters. A good friend was quite visible in his exploits and was able to woo more women in a year than most of our peers had in their lifetime. But we'll be damned if he wasn't the sweetest, most respectful, kind-hearted guy. Like if Michael Buble were cast as Don Draper.

He was a loyal friend and a gentleman, so gossip would come and go but never tarnish his reputation. The adage that will oft be quoted to you in med school regarding social interaction and that especially becomes important when you start clinicals and apply to residency is "don't be an asshole." It doesn't matter how saintly your behavior or how breathtakingly talented you are, if you're an asshole you will get burned.

Finally, don't throw shade. Throughout your career, talking ill of your peers will only ever earn you a poor reputation.

Tips & Tricks from Recent Survivors:

- If you find someone in your class that you are interested in pursuing a serious relationship with, we encourage you to pursue that. But if you're looking to hook up with someone, find someone that doesn't go to your school preferably. Even if you don't talk about it, it isn't certain that the other person will stay quiet too. It is better to avoid that drama all together by finding hook ups outside of your class.

- The dating field can be discouraging for anyone, but it can be especially difficult for women in a high-status profession. It is important to remember to keep high standards and not settle for people who don't appreciate your profession and work.

- <u>Although you may want to keep this part of your life more hidden from your friends in your class, remember to stay safe.</u>

Section 9 – For The Men: What Girlfriend?

You have a girlfriend/boyfriend and you're in medical school? Are you crazy? Yep, you'll hear this a lot.

While they can be an integral part of your support system, a girlfriend can also be a major drain on your time.

The most important thing is establishing ahead of time that school is going to be more important priority than your partnership, at least for the time being. If you are a person who values your family and relationship above everything else, this will be a hard transition. Otherwise, all the time you've sacrificed up to this point will be lost.

That doesn't mean you can't make time for them as well. You just need to be more diligent and schedule your time efficiently. Date night may be a priority this week, but next week you have exams, so date night won't happen. If your anniversary is the same day as your anatomy final, plan for either an early celebration with your partner or plan to skip the post-exam party and go home. The key is that your partner *needs to be on the same page.* Be very careful, a distracting or leeching significant other can quickly drain you of your desire to do any work.

Mark: My girlfriend and I got together early in my first year of medical school and, truth be told, it was amazing. It can be pretty helpful having someone who is essentially contractually obligated to be there for you. This gives a pre-provided shoulder to cry on, which will come in handy after you feel like you failed...Every. Single. Exam. This is also handy on all those days that you feel completely and totally alone in the world and you have someone around to tell you otherwise.

As we said in the last chapters, some of you will be fortunate enough to find your one and only during this time, and this will go on to provide you with many years of happiness. Being able to find someone who understands the strains of medical school and can support you through this is invaluable. For some, this can only be found with someone who is in the same field, or at least in Medicine. For others, finding a grounding, loving partner removed from medicine may be better.

Regardless of their training or background, the key will be the same with any relationship: communication. Every person needs to know that they're loved, even if at the moment you're more intimate with your micro book than your significant other. Take time for the little things. Call them during your five-minute study break. And don't forget birthdays. *Never* forget birthdays.

Chapter 4: Budgeting – How To Spend All The Money That You Don't Have

Section 10 – Make A Budget Already

Budgeting is always and will always be essential. You, like all of us, are on a ten-year journey. And you are going to be very broke for the next ten years through medical school and residency. Get ready for it now. Find cheap food and groceries. Limit your extra drinking. Don't buy that fancy motorcycle you've been eyeing. Or write a book about surviving medical school for extra income...

At some point, almost every physician invests in a financial advisor. This is because eventually you will be making more money than you know what to do with and are going to need help managing it. Not everyone has the option, but if you have the opportunity to develop a relationship with an advisor now, it will help you a lot down the road. In our experience, many will be willing to help you and advise you now for free, with the expectation that someday down the road you will be using their services once you have the money to do so.

Mark: It never hurts to think about the future and plan. It's not typical, but I've had friends in medical school who began investing their extra change, and by residency it's turned into a pretty penny. Again, I'm not the source for how to invest, but if you start early it can add up quickly. Trust me, you'll appreciate all the extra income you can get while in residency.

Missy: I came into med school with the benefit of having worked for the year before, giving me the benefit of a small savings and some practice of living on a budget. Unfortunately, I had to move my sister in with me rent-free for the first two years, replace a totaled car, and cover some untimely hospital fees early on in medical school. If your parents are financially stable, that can be a huge benefit when facing the prospect of being the most destitute and indebted you have ever been in your life. A little bit of a financial safety net goes a long way when unforeseen financial trouble comes up. That was not the case for me, so here's how I set myself up to get through it, and still have enough to spend on leisure activities for my sanity. In case you are wondering, what follows in these chapters is not a coupon-clipping how-to, or being the thriftiest money-saving superstar that can pay off their loans in the first 5 years out of school. Frankly, that kind of thrifty expertise takes a lot of time, which I did not have. But you have a brain, which got you this far, so use it!

If you think you can make a full budget and stick to it, there are plenty of resources out there. Free apps, like like GoodBudget, EveryDollar, or even just using Excel are great ways to start. You Need A

Budget (YNAB) is free for the first year for students and is also an excellent budgeting app. We suggested finding one that works with your needs and then sticking with it.

If you know that you can't stick to a budget, or maybe you're reading this and already don't have the time to commit to make a budget, the easiest way to start controlling your spending is by paying yourself. Put all your money into your savings account or a second checking account. Set up weekly/bi-weekly/monthly "pay days" where you transfer over an amount to your checking. When you run out of that money, you're done until your next pay check comes in. This is by far the most straightforward way to stop spending so much.

Another easy way to motivate you to spend less it to find out how much everything your buying on loans is *actually* costing you. You may buy a $5 coffee now on loan money, but how much will $5 actually be in 4 years after it has gained interest? This is an incredibly sobering way to stop spending money. By looking at your interest rate, you should be able to roughly calculate what you have to multiply things by to find the real cost (ours was around 1.3).

Section 11 - I Need To Check Out These 300 Books, Please

One of the most expensive costs for everyone going through medical school, and any school in fact, is the cost of textbooks. Still stuck in the middle ages of education, many institutions will still require you to purchase books for your courses. However, if you can get around this you should. It is almost guaranteed that there is an upper level somewhere in your school who has found an online version of the textbook. We would never (ahem) never suggest online piracy. But borrowing from someone who has purchased one is perfectly legal.

A much better, and more ethical strategy would be to explore the resources provided to you by your school. In our own institution, the library offered older versions of both print and online textbooks for free. This meant if anyone was willing to take the walk to the library they could get all of their resources for free. This was a common strategy of our second years, who had discovered that buying all the textbooks simply didn't make financial sense. However, having older versions can sometimes put you slightly behind. Be sure your professor isn't using or requiring the most current edition, or you could fall behind. For the majority of cases, though, older editions are just fine to learn the essential information.

If you find you are doing all your studying in the library anyway to get ahold of those books, consider seeing if your school has part-time work study options that will allow you to work at the library desk. You get the benefit of access to all the reserve books while you are on shift, plus you get paid. Your only inconvenience is occasionally checking out or in books for your peers or a possible library catalog search. Wicked easy.

Tips & Tricks From Recent Survivors:

- Unless there is a book that you absolutely love and want in your medical library forever, don't waste a penny on it. Any book that is worth reading will be available somewhere for free. Most of the resources you will need are online subscriptions – Pathoma, Sketchy, Board & Beyond, Uworld, etc.
- There are always ways to get access to subscription content for free. If that goes against your ethical standards, here are some legal ways to cut down on subscription pricing:
    - Group Discounts: most of the time these have been set up beforehand by people before you, but definitely set up group purchases that often cut down on the price
    - Ambassador Programs: some sites (like Sketchy) offer ambassador programs where you can get a free subscription in exchange for posting on Instagram, setting up group orders, or handing out merchandise for your school.
    - Sharing Accounts: some subscription sites allow multiple users on one account while others specifically request you do not do that. Check with older students: sometimes older students will have subscriptions with a couple months left on them that they don't need. You can ask them if you can use it for a couple months. This is particularly helpful if they have questions banks that can be reset.

Section 12 - Top Ramen Is My B*tch

Future doctor's gotta eat. Here's how to save a little and not starve.

1. ***Join every club:*** We say this somewhat facetiously, but the truth is that most academic clubs are eager to attract new members and have a school-sanctioned budget to encourage participation. That translates to plenty of free pizza or subs at the beginning of every academic year. While you may not be interested in becoming a pediatric anesthesiologist, if you're looking for a free meal, going to a meeting is not a bad way to do it. It is also a great way to meet your peers. Who knows, maybe you *will* end up wanting to do Sports Medicine.

2. ***Make friends (especially with people who can cook):*** One of our good friends from med school is a fabulous chef. She loves to cook, and she cooks a lot. Her cooking became a part of our study sessions. The rest of us would make Powerpoint Histology slides, or draw out pathways, and she would feed everyone amazing food. Just don't get selfish. Make sure you're a good friend in return, 'cuz no one likes a mooch.

3. ***Find out where the locals shop:*** When you're new to an area, chances are you will buy groceries at wherever is closest. If that place is Whole Paycheck, then your food money runs out fast. So, talk to the school janitor, the cafeteria worker, the bus driver, the barista, your neighbor walking

their dog, and ask where the best grocery stores are. We were able to find two grocers in Chinatown nearby where we could by 3 bags of produce for under $10. We also learned that the cheapest place to buy most groceries was actually a 5-minute drive from the med school campus, and you could get 3 dozen eggs for 3 dollars.

4. ***Park free:*** Because renting a parking spot is expensive, and don't do it unless you absolutely have to. The biggest tip is this: If you're in a city, look up the parking regulations on the municipal site. You can learn (a) what time parking is free your area, (b) what holidays have free parking, (c) which lots near you are cheapest if you have to park for a day, and (d) if there are parking specials during certain times of the year. Did you know Philadelphia offers free metered parking every Saturday after 11 AM from Thanksgiving until New Years? We didn't either, until we checked their site.

5. ***Take public transit (where applicable):*** This goes with the above in that having a car is expensive. Depending on your school's location, a vehicle may not be necessary before your clinical years. During your clinical years, most schools ship you off to rotations around the state (or in neighboring states) and having a car may be more beneficial. In the pre-clinical years, you can sometimes get away with borrowing a friend's vehicle, renting a car, or using an hourly/daily service like Zipcar or Car-2-Go. Some of us had a vehicle coming in, but it wasn't always cost effective to use it. And it DEFINITELY wasn't cost effective to rely on taxis, Lyft, or Uber to get downtown. Not all public transit is equal. In our experience, rail systems often have the most reliable schedules (the Philadelphia Regional Rail is an exclusive mode of transport through downtown for that reason) and again, the locals will know what is best to take. One of us also got some good insight into what was *safe* to take, with the comment "White girl, you can't go there on the bus!"

6. ***Buy wholesale:*** If you are near a Costco or BJ's or similar wholesale club, we strongly suggest finding a friend and splitting a membership or finding a friend with a membership and going with them whenever they go. Buying your toiletries and frozen food in bulk is the way to go. You'll spend a lot of money at once (we can never seem to spend less than $100 dollars there), but the stuff lasts, and the value is worth it. Another great place to get wholesale prices is to find a grocery store with a bulk foods section. We also suggest learning to love rice. Cheap, easy, and it sustains billions worldwide.

7. ***Learn to cook and get a crockpot:*** The latter is easier than the former. Also, the goal is not to be Top Chef. Making your own food and eating your leftovers is cheaper than eating out. Period. There are tools that can help you with your cooking. The crock pot is a favorite. You can take tough or low-quality meat and slow cook for maximal tenderness. Even if you don't like dark meat chicken, it's cheaper and tastes awesome after a slow cook. You can find lots of recipes online for spices that will make your food taste amazing. You can find cheap spices at places like

Walmart, WinCo (or any grocery store that sells "bulk" spices) and in the "Mexican" or "Latin" section of most grocery stores. Even if you don't speak Spanish, the little plastic packages of garlic and cumin are labeled in English as well. The best part of the crock pot, though, is that you can put everything in the pot before you go to class, turn it on, and when you come home your dinner will be ready. If you like to sleep in, the crock is removable from the heater on most models and you can prep the ingredients the night before and store it in the fridge until the morning. Just remember to take it out of the fridge and turn the heater on the next morning.

8. ***Socialize during happy hour:*** In the pre-clinical years, you will actually have a schedule conducive to an occasional happy hour. If you pick the bar correctly, your dollar can go a long way on wings, sliders, fries, and beer. Not always the healthiest, but your wallet loves it way more than locally sourced sushi. You are also answering the question of "how do I go out on a budget?" Some bars do pub trivia nights with similar specials. Your friends will love that you suggested the break from the books. You will love that you are winning finances.

9. ***Grocery Pick-Up:*** This can save you so much money because it allows you to choose exactly what you need and not be tempted to buy other stuff that will probably just go bad anyway. There are plenty of free grocery pick up options available and some of them can be linked up to coupon apps like iBotta for maximal saving.

Section 13 - Where Did All My Money Go?

Sometimes you didn't budget properly. Sometimes something really shitty happened and your expenses have just tripled. And sometimes, if you're clever, you just want to know your current financial status. Whatever the reason it is to prompt it, we're telling you to go to the financial aid office.

Unless you're an inaccessibly wealthy dragon in the Lonely Mountain, you probably don't have the kind of coin needed to pay for medical school outright. You are going to get a loan. If you are in the military or have joined for medical school, they can help with some loan repayment and unforeseen expenses. For the rest of us civilians, our first go-to in dealing with our loans is the school financial aid office. The lovely staff can help you assess your current loan status, help you adjust your loans if you've come into money, or help you find ways to cover unexpected costs. They often have tricks to readjust your tuition costs if, say, you need another $1500 for the term to cover medical expenses or fly home for a family emergency or just pay rent. Turns out, your itemized medical school expenses cover some things that you don't always need, and a few hundred dollars can often be shifted in a pinch if you are under duress. Some institutions have special scholarships available if you know who or how to ask. Sometimes there are work study opportunities you didn't know about. It is always good practice to chat with the financial aid folks at least once a year to know if things have changed with your loans and make sure your money (or lack thereof) is in the order you expect. Our office also had candy. Sweet.

Your financial aid office may also be able to tell you about scholarships and internship programs that can give you some extra cash. There are usually at least a handful of internships in the anatomy lab or SIM center that can help you bring in an extra penny. On top of that, these look great on your resume and usually allow you the opportunity to develop a closer working relationship with the professors involved.

Many schools also offer tutoring programs where you can get paid to teach a class that you already need to study for! How awesome is that? One of our friends learned best by making study guides. She figured out early on that she could send in the study guides and count them as tutoring hours. Since she was already going to make them, it was no extra time on her part, but she did get paid for them.

Another gig that you can pick up during medical school is house sitting. This is easiest to do if you have connections in the community, but you can sometimes find them through school, too. These are ideal because it normally gives you a quiet place to study—and you're getting paid.

There are some jobs that you can pick up that require a bit more time but can still be worth it. Dog-sitting or grocery-shopping are good ways to take a break from school, earn some money, and get active. Of course, always make sure that you are only doing stuff like this when it will not sacrifice your schoolwork. These kinds of opportunities should always be supplementary during slow weeks and off times, not something that takes away from your studying.

Chapter 5: Some General Advice From Over-achievers About How To Pass Your Classes

This is the section where we try to get a little more specific about the classes you'll take during first year. The obvious difficulty with this is that each school differs greatly in which classes they offer first year. We did our best to offer the most general advice. But since we came from a particular school that did it a particular way, that's how we're going to give it to you. So tough luck.

Section 14 - Anatomy

Anatomy is the crux of medical school. It's why you started in the first place. It's the core of understanding the human body and how it works (*Mark: can you tell this was my favorite subject?*).

When conferring with colleagues throughout our careers, we agree that a solid foundation in anatomy is what has been the most beneficial, second only to pathophysiology in some cases. That being said, to understand Pathophysiology, often Anatomy is necessary. To understand what a problem might be, it's important to understand where it is the way in which it exists. When a patient complains of right upper quadrant pain, you need to know everything that could be the cause so that you can rule them out one by one.

Fortunately, or unfortunately, your anatomy class will likely teach you the information that you'll need to know as a physician, and then multiply it by a factor of 10. Truthfully, other than orthopedist and sports medicine specialists, there are very few physicians who need a thorough knowledge of every muscle in the forearm (which yes, you will be expected to regurgitate). However, this is not the purpose. As with most of the subjects that you learn and then forget, much of what you do retain is worthwhile. For instance, it's always helpful in the ER to understand that the ligaments in the hand are top and bottom in order to be clued into when someone has injured one.

As far as passing the class itself, this is perhaps the most visual of the subjects during your first year. You need to understand where each part exists in space, as well as be able to understand the ridiculous Latin derivative of every body part.

Mark: For me, I found that this came from two things: physical repetition and drawing. Personally, I found that drawing out structures helped me appreciate their relationship to each other. It also helped me slow it down and memorize the names. Netter cards are beautiful, but taking the time to draw out the insertion point of a muscle will help you remember it better than looking at a named blue muscle body (and yes, practical labs will quiz you on what a muscle connects to or how it functions and not just the name).

As far as repetition goes: if you have a cadaver lab, go there. There's no replacement for physically seeing each structure and identifying it. You need to spend as much time with the actual material as possible in order to memorize it. This is also practical as a physician, as you will need to understand the anatomy in real time on a real person when you're caring for them.

Missy: Most of the questions on your practical exam will be on the cadavers that you and your classmates have dissected. Familiarize yourself with each cadaver. If you hear in class, "this is a good example of______" I want you to leave your station and go look at that. As a second year I helped my anatomy professor tag cadavers for the practical exam, and invariably we used the best examples from student dissections that the professor had already identified in class. When we went to grade the practical, the students who did the best were those that I had seen in the lab multiple evenings, looking at cadavers other than their own. Just like your actual future patients, no two bodies are identical and learning the variation is your key to success.

Tips & Tricks from Recent Survivors:

- Anatomy lab is the coolest experience you will get the first two years of medical school. Immersing yourself in anatomy lab not only gives you awesome, slightly sociopathic fodder for conversation starters ("Have you ever sawed a human in half?"), it also gives you memories that will help you get questions right in every other part of medical school and, most importantly, boards. You should be elbow deep in lab every time you go in. Make the most of it.

- It can be overwhelming to go through your first pass with a group of people. You may find it easier to take time to study the material by yourself (or with just one other person) and then incorporate your study group during your second pass of the material.

- If you can't draw but want that visual/tactile association, buy a Netter's anatomy coloring book. They cost around $30 on Amazon and have high yield facts next to each drawing.

- Complete Anatomy and Human Anatomy are great apps to utilize. They have features that allow you to visualize various anatomy structures from the comforts of your own home. They also have clinical sections that gives you a visual run through of various scenarios such as torn ligaments. Complete anatomy was a favorite because of the AR feature.

- When you are reviewing structures, map them out and make connections between them. Tying structures into a bigger system helps you remember where things go and give you a more complete picture of the anatomy. This is particularly helpful as you follow vasculature.

- The time you devote to anatomy lab and the cadaver directly correlates to your anatomy lecture exam grades. Visualizing the structures in person and mapping them out in your head will help you learn the material quicker and more efficiently when studying your lecture slides.

Section 15 – Histology

Most similar to Anatomy, Histology is a very visual field. Perhaps even more so than the former, it relies heavily on your ability to visually recognize an object and then tell everything from it. For this we go back to the same advice: draw it out. By drawing you simultaneously activate two parts of your brain: visual and tactile. This reinforces the material so that it will stick in your brain.

Missy: Now not everyone can be an artist, and some of those cell combinations are a lot harder to draw than a rough sketch of those muscle groups or organs the way you can with anatomy. So, the next best option is print a picture and make flashcards, or better yet do what I did and make a study PowerPoint. Cutting and pasting images from the class PowerPoints (sometimes pausing lectures to screenshot them) and using our library's slide deck (many med schools have digital histology slides you can use) I would make PowerPoints for each exam. The main slide would be the image with the description in the notes section. I would get together with classmates and we would pull the PowerPoint up on a computer or TV screen and quiz each other on cell type, function, etc. It was fun, and also took me significantly less time than drawing. Our pathology teacher once compared finding cells in histo slides to Where's Waldo. For me, gamifying the material with my own slides turned histology into an easy A.

Another major strategy is categorization. It's common sense: it's harder for your brain to memorize ten things than five. So, find a way to group things in your mind. It can be any way that works. Is it easier to remember all the purple stuff together (never try the purple stuff). Or can you group things by type? The more that you can divide things into categories the less daunting the task of memorization will be.

<u>A lot of Histology will be identifying pictures, but a lot of it is also being able to pick out buzz words related to certain slides. If you hear owl eye, you better be thinking Hodgkin Lymphoma. Those are easy points. Unfortunately, boards (and professors) are moving away from buzz words, so you also have to be able to pick through the lengthy, wordy descriptions to figure out what it is they want.</u>

Section 16 - Embryology

There's a reason we started with these first three together. That's because they tend to go hand in hand. These are the most visual of the subjects that you will learn, and they tend to complement each other. As you distinguish between the different branchial clefts, the head and neck anatomy comes into focus. You can see how everything derives from the original embryology, and molds into the human being that we have come here to study. (Ok, maybe it's just me, but I love the continuity.) Because of the continuity, Embryology is particularly helpful to create a timeline for.

Mark: Embryology, more than the preceding two subjects, is all about progression. It's a process, and you need to understand it in the context of time. My personal preference for this particular subject was to tell it as a story. A baby is born, and grows, etc. etc. Take it through each step of the process and tell yourself the story. And don't be afraid to add the hysterical and outrageous. Make your own story that sticks in your mind.

Missy: I liked videos to help me understand these concepts. Guess what? There are hundreds of animations out there. Even YouTube has an embryology channel with legitimate uploads. Many medical schools will have their own sites to link to, but if not, some medical schools offer their videos free online with a simple search.

Chapter 17 – Neuroanatomy

Anatomy. Enough said.

Just kidding.

Neuroanatomy requires the same basic spatial understanding, although it's slightly harder to visualize. While the brain itself may be relatively straightforward and make geographical sense, the neurologic pathways will not. A lot of these are complicated and convoluted, with multiple twists and turns. This will take a lot of repetition and practice to memorize.

For some, this can come naturally as many of the pathways will make sense once you understand them. They also can all be mapped back to their respective areas in the brain. Whatever works for you, writing the pathway out, color-coding areas of the brain to certain pathways on cross-section images, or making a mnemonic, find what works for you.

Not to be taken lightly, Neuroanatomy is one of the more important topics you can master when it comes to being a physician. It seems as though almost every patient has some sort of pain complaint, and understanding the pain pathways, the different dermatomes, and the effects of different stimuli can dramatically improve your diagnostic skills. I know we say this about every subject (because it's true), but this one is valuable to master as a future physician.

Section 18 – Biochemistry

This brings us to one of the more complicated first-year subjects. This particular subject relies on understanding, not just rote memorization. In this it's important to understand your basic organic and inorganic chemistry so you can understand how chemicals operate with each other.

The beautiful thing about Biochemistry is that it follows rules (unlike a lot of the Medicine you'll learn later). Chemistry is based on Physics which is based on Mathematics. Which means that it's predictable. If you can understand the relationships substances have with each other, this becomes simpler.

Now, that doesn't mean that there isn't any memorization. There are plenty of biological systems to learn in which the processes don't make the most sense. You need to learn the different proteins and cellular systems and how they interact.

Mark: Unfortunately (for me) this one, while still visual, is a little more difficult to draw than the former chapters. While you can and should draw out the pathways, it's more about names and arrows that simple pictures. Which means you need to memorize things in terms of pathways instead of as a large picture.

Section 19 - Immunology

This subject is something of a combination between Biochemistry and Histology. There will be a collection of complicated pathways involving the cells and their processes, but also parts of the immune system that require visual memory to understand.

Missy: So this was one where I definitely took advantage of my drawing skills and made flashcards of cells and linking proteins like crazy. Our instructor had gone to the trouble of drawing out cell-to-cell interactions, so I broke those down into easy to associate groups and copied them. Each flash card was a different step in each pathway, so once I learned the steps, I would shuffle them and rearrange them to memorize the order.

As stated, the key with Immunology, as well as some of the more pathway-focused subjects, is understanding the steps. Everything happens in a pre-determined order, and in order to have true understanding your need to know how we get from one step to the next.

Section 20 - Physiology

Many would call this the true heart of Medicine. This is the understanding of how the different systems work within the human body, and it will be truly essential to the rest of your career. As loathe as we are to say it (being Anatomy buffs as we are), this is probably the most important subject to your career in Medicine. A good understanding of Physiology will allow you to solve the most difficult diagnostic dilemmas and give you true understanding of disease and cure.

As such, Physiology is notoriously difficult to learn. A combination of physical and abstract ideas, how do you visualize the fraction of ejected blood with each systolic contraction? This subject thus becomes more of a conglomeration of the physical anatomy that you have learned and Mathematical understanding of systems. Much of Physiology boils down to mathematical equations between systems, and the more right brained people in the room will be drawn to it.

Mark: Don't be discouraged if this doesn't come to you naturally: it's difficult, and something that I still find myself working to master. I would argue that many of my attendings are still working to master this. Only the very few true master diagnosticians have a thorough understanding of human physiology. If you want to be counted among them, then this is your goal.

As with anything, it just takes time and effort. My major recommendation with physiology is to make sure you understand one part before moving onto the next. Many lecturers will present you with pieces of the Physiology picture. However, it's important to understand each system as a whole. Poor understanding of a single part can give a poor groundwork, which will ultimately fall. Don't move onto the next piece until you truly understand the first. Let each piece build on each other.

Missy: This is where having a core study group can really help. To make sure we understood the pathways, my study buddies and I would talk it out, and sometimes take turns drawing it out on whiteboards in our classrooms. Explain one step, pass the baton (or marker) to the next person, they explain a step, and around it goes. Again, if you or someone doesn't understand a step, take the time to stop and break it down. Your friends may have helpful mnemonics to use, or have a better grasp of cardiac physiology, or have been a nephron in their previous life and REALLY know the deal with that loop of Henle.

Section 21 – Additional Resources

There will always be more resources than you will be able to get your hands on. When deciding what resources to use, make sure you choose things that will work for you personally, your studying, and how you think. There are no "best" resources only what is best for you. In order to determine what works for you, ask people who already have resources if you can watch a couple videos on their account (a lot of resources also have sample videos available on YouTube or free trials).

Before you purchase any materials, check with upperclassmen to see if your school has a drive with any resources. On top of outside resources, these drives also usually have study guides for your specific school that can be incredibly helpful. In order to get access to materials like this, you've got to make some good connections with the students above you.

With that being said, here are a handful of resources that we found were incredibly helpful for a majority of our friends in school:

- Osmosis: Osmosis is a subscription based content review course with short, animated videos covering most topics that you will encounter during your curriculum. While the content review aspect is awesome, we think the most helpful feature Osmosis offers is all the practice questions. And the best part is, Osmosis is free if you just want to do the questions! The site offers its own question banks, but individual users can also create question banks – so check to see if older students from your school have practice questions specific to your classes.

- Sketchy: this is an invaluable resource that we cannot recommend enough. We essentially only used this for microbiology and it is close to all you need for pharmacology. Sketchy is essentially a collection of cartoon videos that go through different topics in incredibly memorable and fun ways. There were some people who didn't love Sketchy at the beginning, but essentially everyone has caved as it has gotten closer to boards. Sketchy is incredibly expensive, so make sure to get a group discount for your class. They also have historically offered an ambassador program where you can get a free subscription if you organize and collect payments for group orders for your class.

- Kenhub: This is an additional resource you can use for histology specifically.

- Pathoma: Pathoma is one of the cheaper options on this list, you can get a 2 year subscription and accompanying textbook for under $100! The videos are short and sweet and truly focus on explaining the *why* behind the pathology. It is worth its weight in gold.

- DirtyMedicine: On the opposite end of the spectrum, DirtyMedicine (free resource on Youtube) does not explain why things happen but does offer fun stories and mnemonics to remember all the crazy things you have to shove into your brain for tests. His videos are usually under 10 minutes and are wonderful if you have a hard time with word associations.

- FirstAid has a lot of mnemonics for memorizing the high yield facts. Make sure to flip through that as you work through lectures.

- If you can't find a mnemonic or story to help you memorize something in FirstAid, there is usually something on forums like Reddit or Studentdoctornetwork that can help.

- NinjaNerd: this man is amazing, all we can say. He breaks down everything from physiology to embryology to pathology to EKGs in simple ways that make you feel like you really get it. This is another resource that gets pretty deep into the *why* behind medicine. Currently, his videos are all free on Youtube.

Section 22 – The Staff

Much of medical school can feel impersonal, but it doesn't have to. All of Medicine is about people and making relationships. There is no better place to start than in your first year with the people you are working with.

If you haven't figured out the game yet, the truth about medical school (and all academia as we see it) just comes down to passing a test. And who creates these tests, who grades them? People. Humans. Professors. The professors that will be teaching you are by far the most important resource for you to access during your studies.

For many medical schools, the classes are large, and the professors are used to being distant with their students. If you can be the one person who changes the paradigm, this puts you at a gigantic advantage. Show the staff that you want to succeed and are willing to do the work, and you will reap the rewards. On top of the staff seeing you differently, when you start seeing that the staff and the institution are not out to get you, it makes the entire medical school experience more enjoyable. It also makes it easier to learn under people when you know and enjoy them.

In medical school, you are working towards earning the same credentials that your professors hold, so they truly are closer to senior colleagues than professors have ever been before. Additionally, most medical school professors see your performance as a direct reflection of their mentorship and are highly invested in your success. Take advantage of this and pursue meaningful friendships with your professors.

Mark: From personal experience, befriending the faculty carries numerous benefits. I myself could be found venting in my dean's office once a week about the stresses of medical school and how I couldn't handle it. Because I had developed a real relationship with my anatomy and micro professors, when I had been dealt an unfair grade by a new professor, they were eager to help.

Missy: My love of Anatomy stemmed from our wonderful professor, who opened his lovely home to me on more than one occasion. When I had appendicitis in medical school, our pathology teacher cut me an extra set of slides of my appendix and went through my pathology with me. Surgery was actually my most frustrating clinical rotation. I had never complained more, I had never felt so unsure of myself, and I could honestly rank the experience near the bottom of my clinical time. But I met my mentor, a talented vascular surgeon who loved to teach, he encouraged me and I never looked back. You will find that the experiences you have with the staff will shape your path through medical school. Your first year is the best time to start developing good relationships and avoid falling into bad ones.

About Us

As a couple gunners and a team of friends who may or may not have struggled intermittently through medical school (did, definitely did), we wanted to find a way to reach out to new medical students and help them as they entered this crucial portion of their life. We also know that we are in the unique situation of having very different approaches to medical school itself.

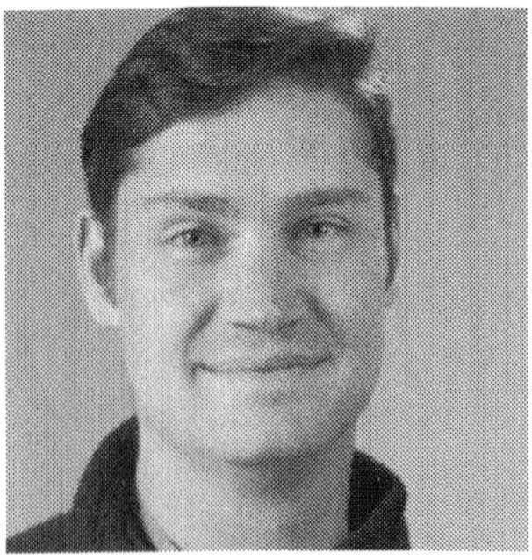

Mark: I was one of those somewhat unlucky individuals who scraped by just enough to get into medical school. While I was resentful of this at first, I soon realized that it gave me the attitude and determination I needed to succeed. For the first few years I worked so hard that my soon to be friends thought I was simply a crazy person to be shunned. Eventually I made lifelong friends like those in this book and returned to being a normal human being. In addition, I had gone from a student barely getting by to one of the top in the class. I don't say this to brag, I for one know my limitations (and let me tell you, they are many), but to inspire. I hope that by hearing my story and learning from my mistakes another underdog like myself can rise to the challenge and be the next great physician.

Dr. Wiseman attended Drexel University College of Medicine in Philadelphia prior to ultimately completing his residency in Emergency Medicine at the same institution in Philadelphia. After obtaining a few years working as an attending during the COVID pandemic he then returned for more training by attending a Surgical Critical Care fellowship at St. Luke's University Hospital in Bethlehem Pennsylvania. Dr. Wiseman is currently a full time faculty member at Houston Memorial Hospital in the Cardiothoracic and Cardiovascular Intensive Care Units where he continues to focus on training physicians of all levels of experience.

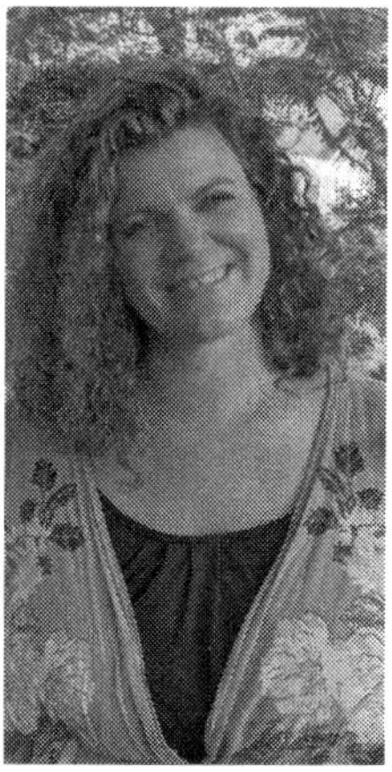

Missy: According to Mark I was one of those "lucky ones" and I have to admit that medical school probably came a bit easier for me than it did for some of my classmates. However, as we say in the book, no one gets through medical school without having to put in the work. I also came to medical school with the perspective of trying to live and study on a pretty strict budget. I came from a pretty poor family who I had to help support, including moving my sister in with me during my first part of medical school. I learned some tricks to help me manage my finances, and they really apply to anyone who's coming in as a medical student. I'm hoping this can make the transition a little easier so you all can struggle a little less than I did.

After completing her medical school education at Drexel University in Philadelphia (where she graduated AOA), Dr. Missy DeSouza moved west to complete surgical residency at Oregon Health and Science University. She went on to complete fellowship training in Foregut Surgery before joining The Oregon Clinic, where she specializes in advanced minimally invasive treatment of esophagogastric disease. She continues to work with trainees across all levels, encouraging growth, research, and passing on the lessons she has learned through her education.

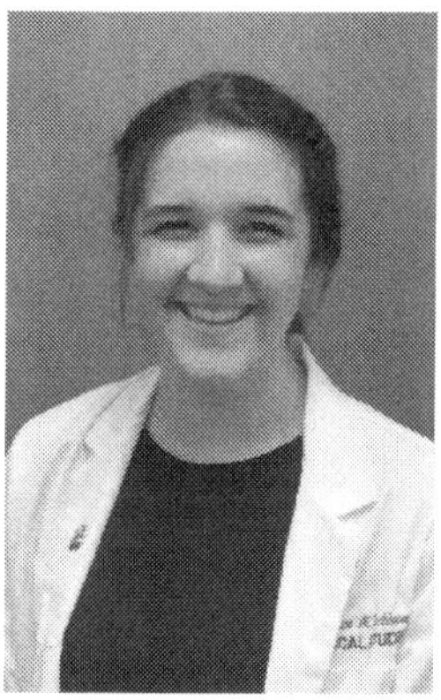

Jessie Barkhouse was born in Greece and raised in the Republic of Kosovo. Fueled by the health disparities witnessed in her community, she decided to become a doctor to provide care to marginalized patient groups. Jessie is completing her medical training at Edward Via College of Osteopathic Medicine in hopes of incorporating the American values of excellence and equality with the Kosovar values of community, rest, and hospitality in her medical practice.

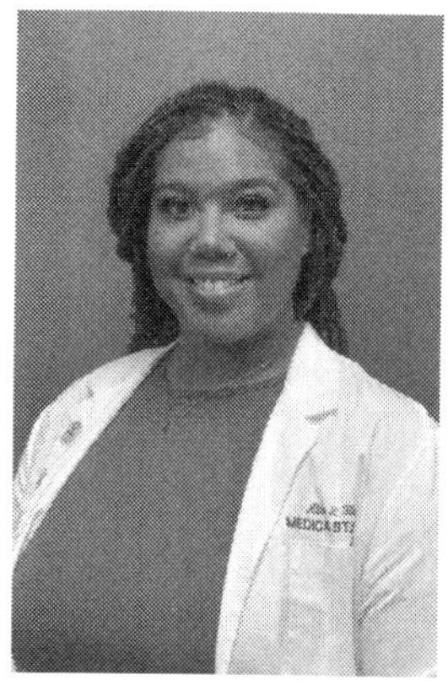

Alisha Tillman is a proud alumnus of Alabama A&M, where she devoted hours to serving her institution through academics and leadership. Ms. Tillman is currently an OMS2 student at Edward Via College of Osteopathic Medicine-Auburn where she serves as a student ambassador, a member of various organizations, and a simulation center research intern. With her dedication to women's health and underserved communities, she recently founded Project Forward, a community health project that provides education and tangible support to post-partum mothers in the local Auburn community. Ms. Tillman hopes to use her medical career to continue serving under-resourced communities.

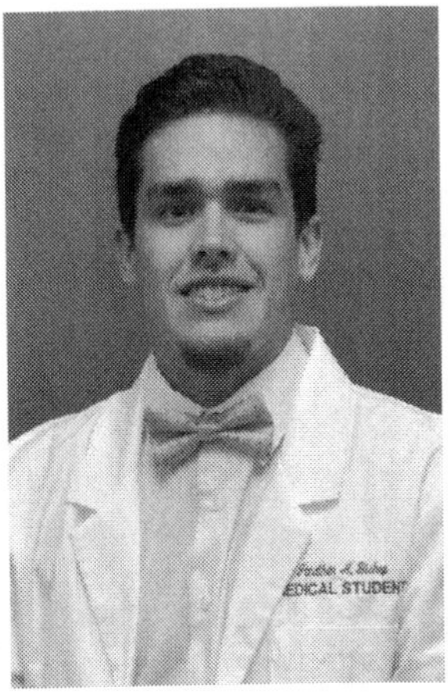

Jonathan Bishop was born in London and grew up in Miami where he completed his undergraduate degree at Florida International University. He is an OMS-2 at Edward Via College of Osteopathic Medicine in Auburn, Alabama. Johnathan is currently the COSGP Global Health Liaison at VCOM Auburn and enjoys working alongside his peers to reach a collective goal. His past experiences as a teacher and coach have instilled the importance of passing on knowledge to future medical students so they can be successful future physicians.

Resources:

1. Peter Densen, MD. Challenges and Opportunities Facing Medical Education. *Trans Am Clin Climatol Associ* 2011;122:48-58.
2. Nauert R PhD. Taking breaks found to improve attention. Psych Central. https://psychcentral.com/news/2011/02/09/taking-breaks-found-to-improve-attention/23329.html
3. Coffield F, Moseley D, Hall E et al. Learning styles and pedagogy in post-16 learning: a systematic and critical review. Learning & Skills research Centre, 2004.
4. Astin JA. Stress reduction through mindfulness meditation, effects on psychological symptomatology, sense of control and spiritual experiences. Psychother Psychosom 1997;66;97-106.

Other Books From The Healthcare Lab, Inc.

In fact, 99.9% error-free is not ok in Healthcare. And in *Ten Secrets*, national quality experts including Malcom Baldrige Award reviewers, Lean Six Sigma Master Black Belts, and practicing healthcare providers share key, high-level information to help get you and your team beyond routine levels of performance...because the patients are worth it.

<u>Games for Health: Ultimate Beginner's Guide To Using Game Dynamics In Healthcare Organizations</u>

Let's make working in healthcare even more fun...and effective!

There's an engagement crisis among healthcare workers...

According to recent reports, 70% of workers are either not engaged in their work or are actively trying to hurt their company. This lack of engagement leads to missed opportunities, revenue problems, and quality issues. One useful solution is the application of game dynamics to your current system and culture--and this work provides the tools to do just that. Use *Games for Health* to apply game dynamics to healthcare settings in order to facilitate culture change, quality improvement, and better patient care!

<u>Trauma Program Operator's Manual</u>

The Practical, Insider's Guide To Running A Trauma Program

The Trauma Program Operator's Manual Gives You Tools To Succeed!

If you're involved with a trauma program in any way, this manual is for you. It's filled with useful, hard to find info that helps guide your trauma program to excellence and beyond!

<u>Healthcare Information System Hacking: Protect Your System</u>

Understand how your health information is at risk and how hackers attempt to obtain it.

Healthcare Information System Hacking tells you specifics about what you need to protect your private health information, whether you're a system administrator, patient, or healthcare provider.

Learn the true value of your health information, and how hackers attempt to access it. *Healthcare Information System Hacking* introduces the specific steps hackers follow to obtain information from a hospital or health system. This book is great for information professionals in healthcare and concerned patients alike!

Made in the USA
Las Vegas, NV
21 July 2026

51328008R00026